I0765617

ABOUT THE AUTHOR

THE AUTHOR OF THIS BOOK, DR.SUDIPTA KR BARMAN IS A NEUROPHYSIOTHERAPIST,PAIN MEDICINE EXPERT AND A CLINICAL NEUTRITIONIST FOR OBESITY CARE.

HE PASSED MASTERS OF PHYSICAL THERAPY IN NEUROSCIENCE FROM A REPUTED UNIVERSITY IN INDIA.HE ALSO GOT POST GRAGUATE DIPLOMA IN PAIN MEDICINE,OBESITY CARE,INFECTIOUS DISEASE,NEUTRITION AND GERIARIATRICS FROM CDC ATLANTA..

HE ALSO HOLDS MANY DEGREES AND CERTIFICATIONS FROM WHO INTERNATIONAL,SUCH AS INCIDENT MANAGEMENT SYSTEM,OCCUPATIONAL HEALTH AND SAFETY,MOTIVATIONAL INTERVIEW WITH

PATIENTS,DISUSTER MANAGEMENT,DISEASE CONTROLE AND PREVENTION.

<u>DEDICATION</u>

THIS BOOK IS DEDICATED TO MY PARENTS (Smt.NITA BARMAN AND Mr.SWAPAN KUMAR BARMAN)

WITHOUT THEIR HELP AND SUPPORT IM JUST NOTHING IN THIS WORLD.

<u>PREFACE</u>

THIS BOOK IS ENTIRELY FOCUSED ON AN UPCOMING GLOBAL EPIDEMIC NAMED   'TEXT NECK DISEASE'.

EACH AND EVERY ASPECT OF THIS HEALTH ISSUE LIKE CAUSE, SYMPTOMS(EARLY AND DELAYED),RISK FACTORS,AGE GROUP INVOLVED,SELF ASSESSMENT,PREVENTION MANAGEMENT ADVICE, ALL ARE EXPLAINED.

THIS BOOK IS DESIGNED FOR EVERY TYPE OF PEOPLE IN THIS SOCIETY.

PLEASE READ CAREFULLY, UNDERSTAND THE ISSUE, ASSESS YOUR SELF FOR SUSCEPTABILITY, EXICUTE THE ADIVICE, AND GIFT YOURSELF A PAIN FREE QUALITY LIFE.

CHAPTER 1

Before starting the discussion of the main topic , I want to share an experience during one of my clinical hours. It's interesting. Read with concentration and try to understand the issue.

One patient came to me with a bunch of reports of a cardiologist, which contains lots of prescriptions and investigations like ecg,echo,tmt,full blood examinations' . I talked with him, what is your problem?

He replies that he is having an occasional irritating chest pain (retrosternal discomfort) from last 1 year. His age is 35yrs.he also included that he consulted all the top cardiologist in the town and done all possible investigations regarding any heart issue, but his heart condition is normal according to the cardio doctors and reports also.

Simply think, how much disturbing is this for a common man?

Then I askd him if he has any kind of headaches or neck pain. He told he used to have an occasional headache but no neck pain.

I ask him to come with a simple x-ray of neck and after getting the x-ray plat I saw a early degeneration of cervical spine with reduced disc space and loss of cervical curvatures.

I told him that you just don't have to worry about your heart but you should concentrate on your neck because the chest pain is the sign of weakness of neck muscle and early degeneration.

I treated his neck for a few days and give some postural advice and exercise. Now he is totally cured.

So just think how important your neck is. Any problem in neck can cause chest pain because of same dermatomal innervations property of nerves.

Do you know neck problems can change your strength of eye sight?

Do you know neck problem can cause VERTIGO AND DIZZINESS?

Do you know nack issue can cause pain in jaw and air sinuses?

Do you know faulty neck can cause difficulty in swallowing difficulty?

Such lots of thing I'm going to discuss in this book related to TEXT NECK DISEASE.

Read carefully whether you have early neck problem or not and try to execute the protocols I will give you for self diagnosis or differential diagnosis of TEXT NECK.

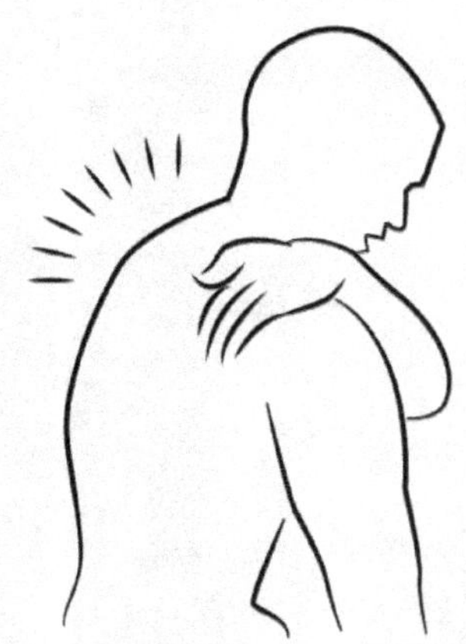

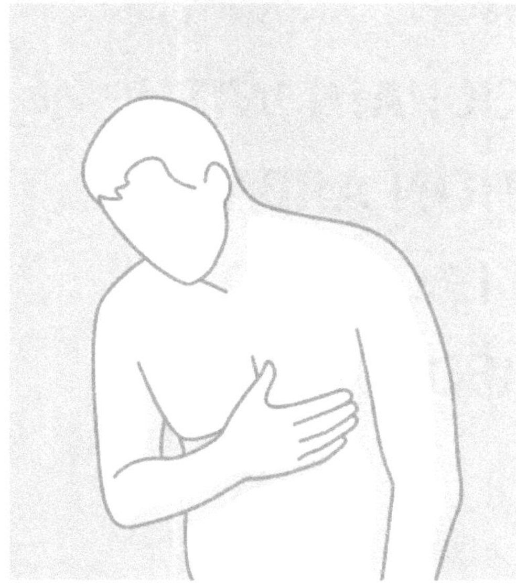

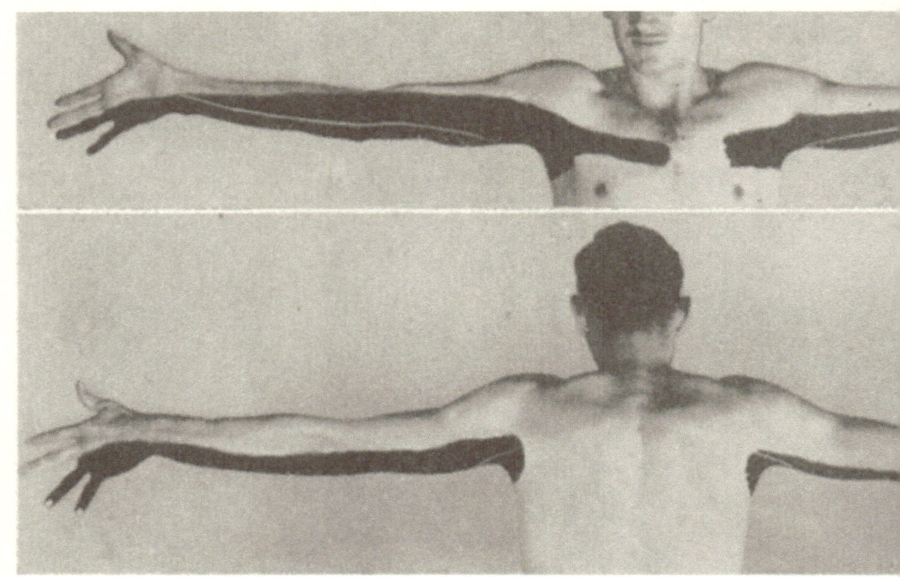

NECK PAIN WITH RADIATION AREAS WHICH IS CALLED REFERRED PAIN

CAPTER 2

ANATOMY OR GROSS STRUCTURE OF YOUR NECK

Compartments:-

The neck structures are distributed within four compartments:

- **Vertebral compartment** contains the cervical vertebrae with cartilaginous discs between each vertebral body. The alignment of the vertebrae defines the shape of the human neck.[5] As the vertebrae bound the spinal canal, the cervical portion of the spinal cord is also found within the neck.

- **Visceral compartment** accommodates the trachea, larynx, pharynx, thyroid and parathyro id glands.

- **Vascular compartment** is paired and consists of the two carotid sheaths found on each side of the trachea. Each carotid sheath contains the vagus nerve, common carotid artery and internal jugular vein.

Besides the listed structures, the neck contains cervical lymph nodes which surround the blood vessels.

Muscles and triangles

Muscles of the neck attach to the skull, hyoid bone, clavicles and the sternum. They bound the two major neck triangles; anterior and posterior.

Anterior triangle is defined by the anterior border of the sternocleidomastoid muscle, inferior edge of the mandible and the midline of the neck. It contains the stylohyoid, digastric, mylohyoid, geniohyoid, omohyoid, sternohyoid, thyrohyoid and sternothyroid muscles. These muscles are grouped as the suprahyoid and infrahyoid muscles depending if they are located superiorly or inferiorly to the hyoid bone. The suprahyoid muscles (stylohyoid, digastric, mylohyoid, geniohyoid) elevate the hyoid bone, while the infrahyoid muscles (omohyoid, sternohyoid, thyrohyoid, sternothyroid) depress it. Acting synchronously, both groups facilitate speech and swallowing. **Posterior triangle** is bordered by the posterior border of the sternocleidomastoid muscle, anterior border of the trapezius muscle and the superior edge of the middle third of the clavicle. This triangle contains the sternocleidomastoid, trapezius, splenius capitis, levator scapulae, omohyoid, anterior, middle and posterior scalene muscles.

Nerve supply

Sensation to the front areas of the neck comes from the roots of the spinal nerves C2-C4, and at the back of the neck from the roots of C4-C5.

In addition to nerves coming from and within the human spine, the accessory nerve and vagus nerve travel down the neck.

Blood supply and vessels

Arteries which supply the neck are common carotid arteries which bifurcate into: - Internal carotid artery - External carotid artery

THIS PAGE KEEPS INTENTIONALLY BLANK

SURFACE ANATOMY OF NECK

The thyroid cartilage of the larynx forms a bulge in the midline of the neck called the Adam's apple. The Adam's apple is usually more prominent in men. Inferior to the Adam's apple is the cricoid cartilage. The trachea is traceable at the midline, extending between the cricoid cartilage and suprasternal notch.

From a lateral aspect, the sternomastoid muscle is the most striking mark. It separates the anterior triangle of the neck from the posterior. The upper part of the anterior triangle contains the submandibular glands, which lie just below the posterior half of the mandible. The line of the common and the external carotid arteries can be marked by joining the sterno-clavicular articulation to the angle of the jaw. Neck lines appear at a later age as a development of skin wrinkles.

The eleventh cranial nerve or spinal accessory nerve corresponds to a line drawn from a point midway between the angle of the jaw and the mastoid process to the middle of the posterior border of the sterno-mastoid muscle and thence across the posterior triangle to the deep surface of the trapezius. The external jugular vein can usually be seen

through the skin; it runs in a line drawn from the angle of the jaw to the middle of the <u>clavicle</u>, and close to it are some small lymphatic glands. The <u>anterior jugular vein</u> is smaller, and runs down about half an inch from the middle line of the neck.
The <u>clavicle</u> or collar-bone forms the lower limit of the neck, and laterally the outward slope of the neck to the shoulder is caused by the <u>trapezius muscle</u>.

The neck is the region between the head and the rest of the body, which is built of different tissue and organs, including many skeletal muscles. The main functions of the **neck muscles** are to permit movements of the neck or head and to provide structural support of the head. The **muscles of the neck** can be divided into groups according to their location.

The **superficial neck muscles** are the most external and include the platysma and the sternocleidomastoid.

The **suprahyoid muscles** are a group of **neck muscles** located above the hyoid bone and all elevate this bone, while the **infrahyoid muscles** are situated below the hyoid bone and participate in depressing it.

The three **scalene muscles** are located in the lateral part of the neck.

The **prevertebral muscles of the neck** are situated anterior to the vertebral column.

In the upper posterior part of the neck below the occipital bone the four paired **suboccipital muscles** are situated. These muscles can also be categorized among the deep muscles of the back.

Several other muscles of the back also extend up to the neck region and are partly connected with the cervical part of the vertebral column, including the trapezius, levator scapulae, splenius, iliocostalis, longissimus, rotatores, semispinalis, interspinales, and intertransversarii muscles.

MOVEMENTS OF NECK

<u>Neck</u> upper (<u>Atlantoccipital</u> & <u>Antlantoaxial</u>) FlexionExtension / HyperextensionLateral Flexion (Abduction)Reduction (Adduction)Rotation

Cervical spine	Flexion	Extension / Hyperextension
	Lateral Flexion (Abduction)	Reduction (Adduction)
	Rotation	
Thoracic spine	Flexion	Extension / Hyperextension
	Lateral Flexion (Abduction)	Reduction (Adduction)
	Rotation	
Lumbar spine	Flexion	Extension / Hyperextension

TEXT NECK DISEASE

	Lateral Flexion (Abduction)	Reduction (Adduction)
	Rotation	

(REFERENCE OR SOURCE IS wekepedia)

Here all movements of spine is given.this are the all essential movements wich normall occurred in your cervical(neck) as well as your full spine.every movement is affected by above and below segmental movements.

<u>TEXT NECK</u>

What is TEXT NECK?

It is a modern era term of early age neck pain with multiple associated symptoms given by an American chiropractor DR.D.L.FISHMAN.

In one word it is a neck-shoulder pain symptom complex.

Causes of TEXT NECK

It is the result of repeated stress and micro injury of neck structures which causes or creates a neck-shoulder pain complex.

Other name of this condition is turtle neck posture or anterior head syndrome. Some important causes are—

1. Constant usage of hand held gadgets like mobile,tab,laptops which directly produce an impact over neck irrespective of your age.

2. Watching TV for a prolonged time without proper posture

3. in appropriate writing desk design for students.

4. Faulty sitting arrangements for an IT professional or corporate worker.

In this modern, fast and rapid growing age, the use of mobile is hiking up day by day all over the world. It is becoming unavoidable. But we don't know the way of proper use of it. So if you don't know or don't want to know then the impact will change your quality of lifestyle entirely.

SYMPTOMS OF TEXT NECK

SEVERAL EARLY SYMPTOMS ARE THERE.

1. Dull aching pain in early stage of disease in the lower part of neck, which may be Sharpe and stabbing type in advanced and extreme conditions.

2. Difficulty in neck movements which is called stiff neck after a usages.

3. Due to this pain and muscle spasm the paraspinal muscles of neck like trapezius,rhomboids got weak. As a result the pain got worse with minimal activity.

4. Due to tightness of sub-occipital muscle group there is a typical tension headache encountered

frequently, which relieved by rest. This pain is like heaviness of back of head and quiet irritating.

5. Morning stiffness, which means a strong spasm present in neck in the morning after rising up from the bed. This usually subsides after few hours with neck movements. Those who having morning stiffness often dislikes soft and high head sleeping pillow.

6. Someone may feel discomfort in holding neck upright in front of computers in office environment after a few hours of usage.

This above are the early signs and symptoms of text neck. But when it becomes chronic it may bring several greater problems like---

1. Thoracic kyphosis or hunch back deformity in back.

2. Early degenerative spondylopathy like osteophytes formation with spondylitis.

3. Inter vertebral disc may gets degeneration due to over or uneven loading.

4. The muscles of neck and shoulder girdle may get atrophied due to prolonged weakness and lack of optimum use.

5. Frozen shoulder with bicipital tendinitis which is very irritating pathological conditions where patient can not lift their arm up due to pain. They often complain that they are getting nocturnal pain in shoulder.

6.spinal canal stenosis which is condition where the space for spinal cord and nerve roots is compromised due to space occupying lesions by disc or osteophytes.here patient can often feel a tingling sensation with numbness and pin in upper limb(unilateral or bilateral)

7. Due to change in the curvature in the spine in nack,where will be reduced capacity of lungs.in one term vital capacity of lungs is reduced

PATHOMECHANICS OF TEXT

How texting could damage your spine

Forces on the neck increase the more we tilt our heads, causing spine curvature

Force on neck	10-12lb	27lb	40lb	49lb	60lb
Neck tilt	0 degrees	15 degrees	30 degrees	45 degrees	60 degrees

NECK

As I have told that cervical spine is a segmental chain of spin which consist of 7 cervical vertebras. These vertebras are separated from each other by intervertebral discs which act like a shock absorber to cervical spine. These two structures are surrounded and supported by several paraspinal muscles and ligaments and fascia. In normal spine the cervical segment got a normal anterior curvature which in term called normal cervical lodosis.

Now see the above picture. When your head is aligned in neutral or upright position, a 10-12 lbs weight is falling on your neck. But when you are starting changing the angulations' of neck then the weight also increasing on neck and if it remains for a long duration very frequently then an obvious change will be there in your neck. And it will cost you. Some changes that might occur in cervical spine in text neck are mentioned before.

Text neck can bring problems in thoracic and lumbar spine also if you do not treat yourself for a long time.

<u>WHO ARE AT GREAT RISK OF TEXT NECK?</u>

Text neck is a life style disease. Which means your life style is the key factor of developing this disorder. Study is saying that within next 2 years every 3 person (child or adult) among 10 people in the world will suffer from TEXT NECK. So who are at a great risk? Check below

1. Young childrens who make mobile and tablets vigorously for gaming, watching videos and don't habit an outdoor sport. Spending time in mobile for hours causes lack of physical activity, inadequate exposure to sunlight, early obesity and faulty neck posture. This factors brings not only text neck but also some serious health issues like fatty liver, severe growth pain, growth disorders, lack of

intelligence,headache,reduced eyesight,dipressive disorders.

So parents, beware .don't let your child to be controlled by mobiles or tablets or pc.

2. Average adults who think that the only to time pass is to make engaged them in social networking sites for nothing. Doing chating,surfing unnecessary things by bending your neck all the free time. When mobile is not there and the internet was not so cheap, maximum of our adult population used to spend their free time by gossiping, reading newspaper, writing some stuffs. They were good. But now a days when get in a train you will see that everyone is busy with their mobiles or tablets. Also the close their ear by ear pods. This how not only text neck is developing, but there is some greater problems are waiting like depression, migraine headache disorders, and mood disorders.

Depression is the mother of all degenerative diseases like arthritis, fibromyalgia.

So this type of folks cannot escape the TEXT NECK and its consequences.

3. Corporate and IT professionals spends their maximum time with their P.C or laptops. This job. you has to do it. But keep in mind that you cannot escape TEXT NECK if you don't change your office ergonomics. You have to take the help of an expert for this.dont just Google and make some self designed ergonomics for yourself. Because in this case you will do more harm to you.

UNAVOIDABLE CONSEQUENCES OF TEXT NECK

If you don't correct or treat yourself or your mobile addicted Childs what are the serious health issues may arise:-

1. Headaches disorders

2. Growth disorders in Childs

3. Hormonal disorders in Childs.

4. Vision problem.

5. Poor IQ in growing Childs

6. Mood and depressive disorders sleep disorders

7. Advanced level spondylopathy like spinal cannel stenosis,prolapsed disk, slippage of vertebra, neural reticular pain etc.

8. Benign postural vertigo

More problems are there, but I just don't want to make everything here in this book. A few should be left for my next books topic…..

Now I'm coming in prevention and treatment of this irritating TEXT NECK PAIN…..

Don't just read it; try to execute it in your life. Then only your money and my efforts will not lose.

<u>HOW TO AVOID TEXT NECK FROM HAPPENING</u>

I'm not telling to drop your mobiles,tabs,laptops. Without them we are blind in this age. Use them in a healthy manner. We, use mobile. So don't just let mobile to use and control us. Here I'm going to talk about the possible things which every should imply in their life to avoid this text neck pain.

1. Just work on yourself for only 30 minutes per day. Here you can do several core exercises or yoga postures or some other form of physical exercises.try to do it in the starting of the day. Because your mind have very deep relation with your health. in morning our mind stays fit and fine. So whatever you do in this time it will be well absorbed by your body and you get the best results. So make it a habit to early rise.

2. Make a schedule for your social networking involvement. Make it in your own way but I should not be more than 5 minutes in a session. You can take maximum7-8 such sessions per day. Design it with your own necessecity. Always

remember, don't be the pet of our digital master (gadgets).

3. Don't allows your child to play with or watch mobiles. Make them understand the actual scientific usages of gadgets from the very beginning of their life. For example make the understand that mobile is the calling device only. You can only talk with someone with it. Don't surf internet or spend time on social media in front of them. Encourage them in outdoor sports.

Impact of mobile in Childs is not only physical; there is very strong negative impact on their mind and intelligence. So keep mobile out of reach of children.

4. Now a day's too many IT professional and corporate workers are facing this TEXT NECK PROBLEM, but they just don't know it's happening because of their unhealthy work patterns and faulty postures which they can correct.

Neck and shoulder complex pain makes their life so irritating that they want to work hard but cant.

Please change you're sitting ergonomics or office ergonomics. For this you can seek help for a physiotherapist. He will explain and design your work environment to prevent text neck. I will also provide some diagram which you can try to apply. It can be helpful.

5. Do some static and dynamic neck and shoulder complex exercise at home regularly. Make it a habit. You will confident and fit.

6. Mental health is directly related with disc degeneration. So always be happy, don't take stress and tension beyond your threshold.

7. You can attain a good yoga studio and learn some good yoga fitness postures.

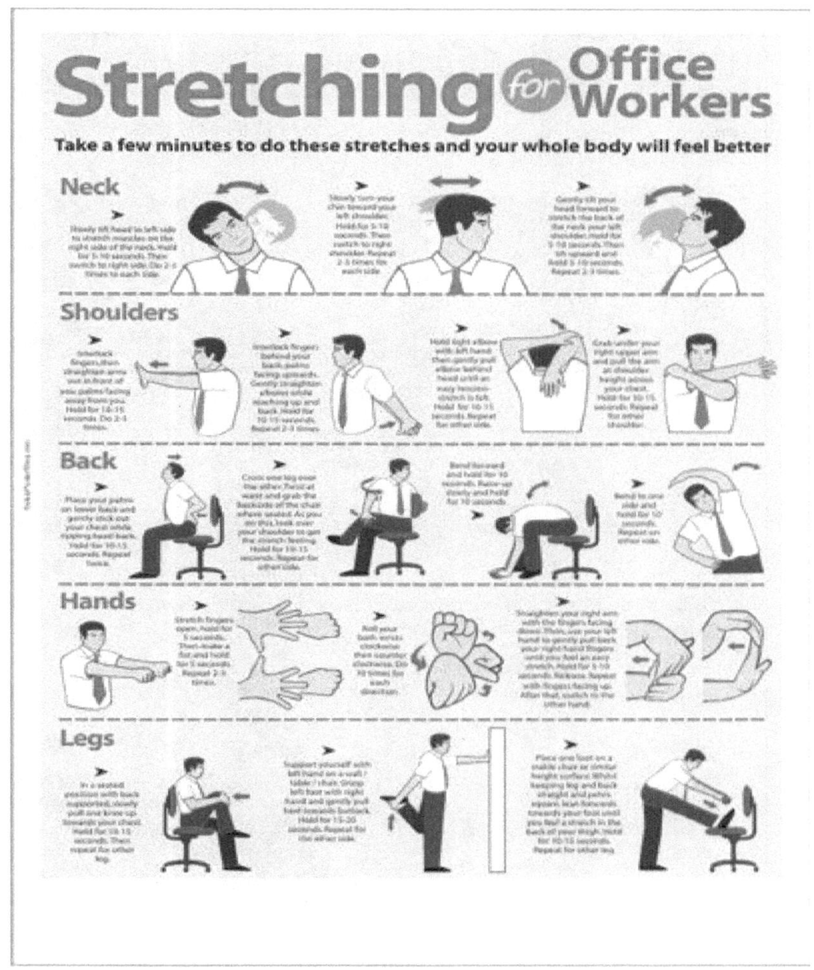

These are the exercise you can do at office easily in between work to keep fitness.

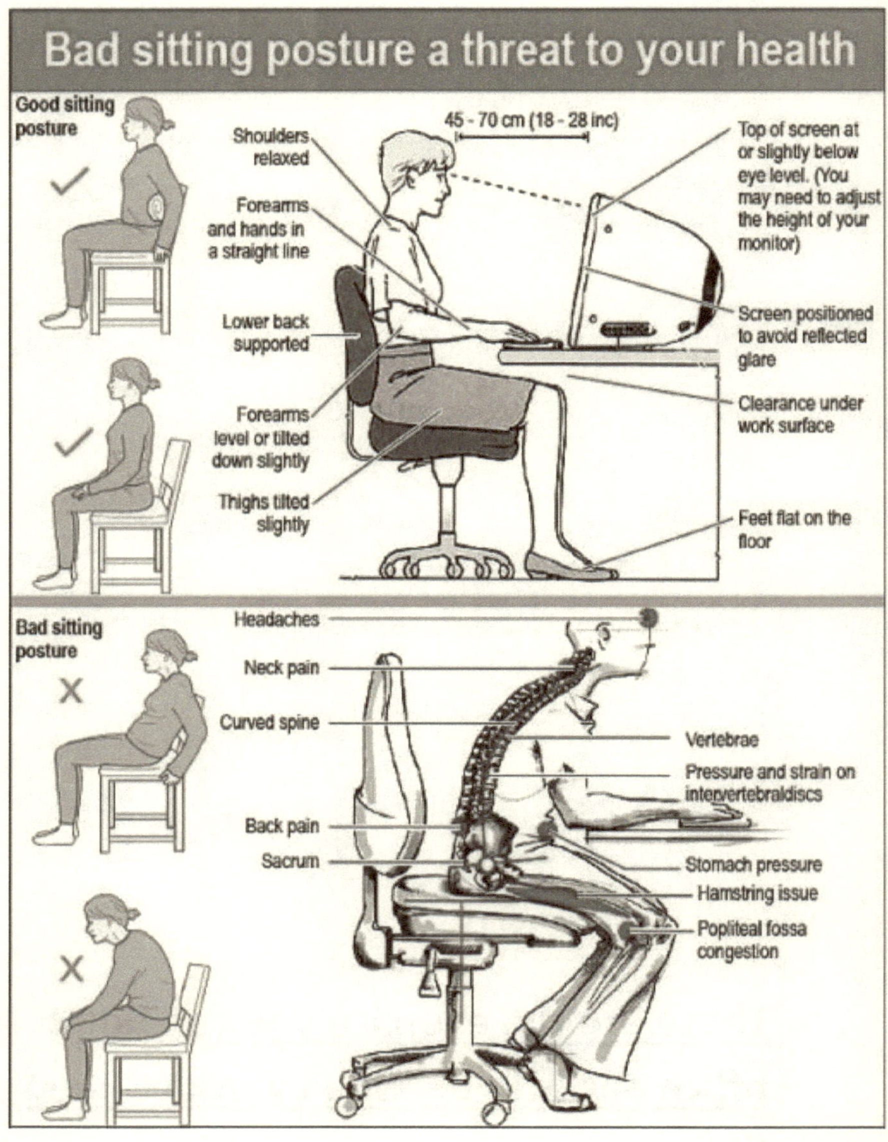

Bad sitting posture a threat to your health
Good sitting posture
Bad sitting posture
Shoulders relaxed
Forearms and hands in a straight line
Lower back supported
Forearms level or tilted down slightly
Thighs tilted slightly
45 - 70 cm (18 - 28 inc)
Top of screen at or slightly below eye level. (You may need to adjust the height of your monitor)
Screen positioned to avoid reflected glare
Clearance under work surface
Feet flat on the floor
Headaches
Neck pain
Curved spine
Back pain
Sacrum
Vertebrae
Pressure and strain on intervertebraldiscs
Stomach pressure
Hamstring issue
Popliteal fossa congestion

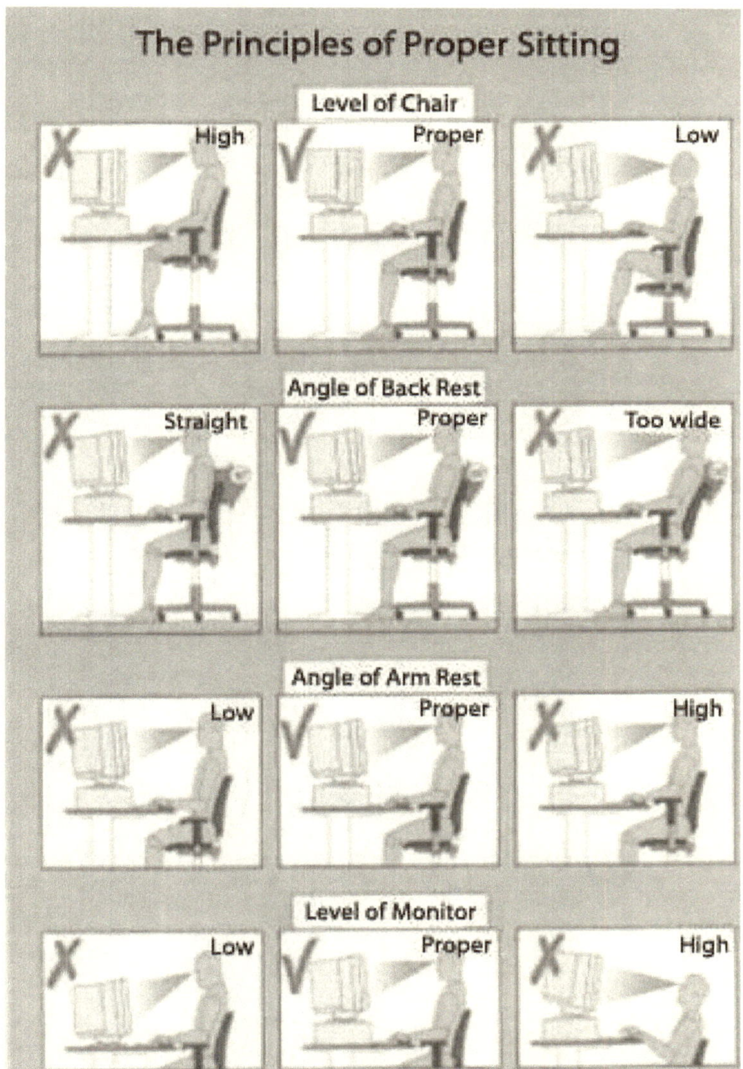

Try to understand this image.

Keep good form with your stand-up desk

Here's what to do if you plan to be on your feet all day

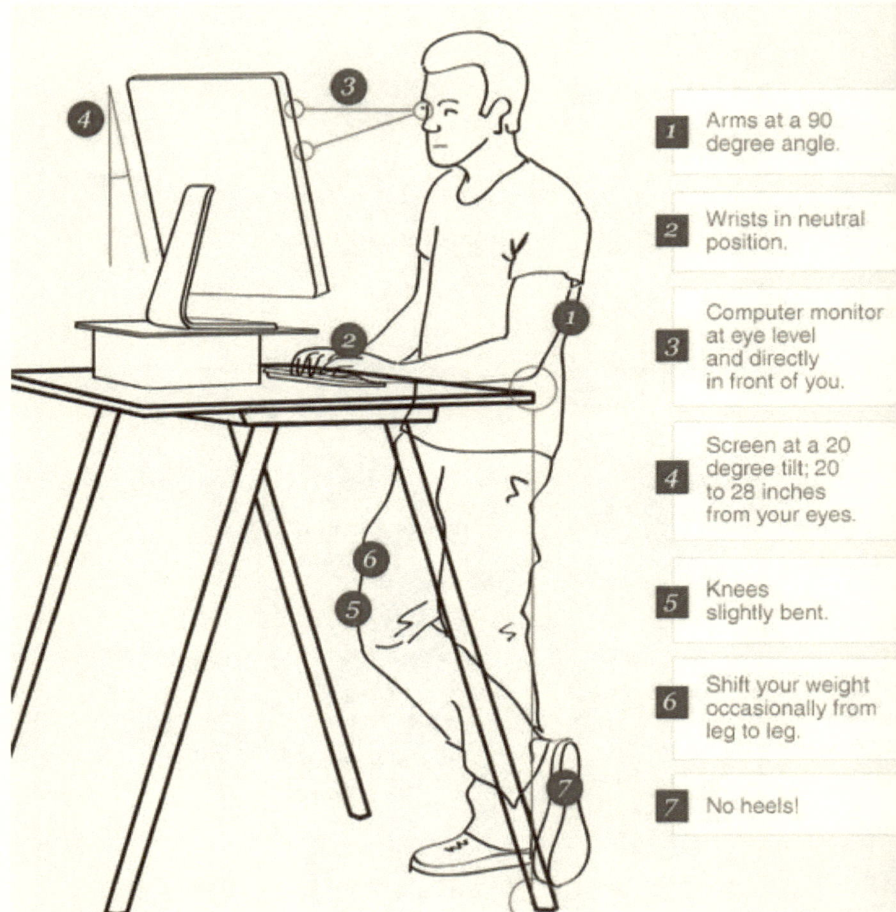

(Picture source printerest)

TREATMENT:-

First I will discuss about the **home treatments**. This is simple and you can do without the help of anyone.

1. Essential oils

Make a blend of extra virgin olive oil with chamomile,lavender,rosemary,marjoram essential oils in 2:1:1:1:1 ratio and keep it in glass container.

Apply this at night by a little massage over neck and shoulders. Your neck muscles will get relaxation and pain will be gone. It will act like a natural pain killer

2.do some neck and shoulder girdle exercise regularly like, static neck isometrics, shoulder rotation, chin tuck exercise, normal all neck movements up to pain free range.

You can do some yoga posture like Bhujangasana,nukasana.

3. Apply ice in summer and hot pack in winter at the affected parts.

4. Buy a cervical memory foam pillow and use it. It will keep your cervical curvature maintained.

5. Sleep in a firm, uniform bed. Avoid soft surface to sleep.

6. Swimming is a great exercise to your spine.

7. Quit alcohol and smocking.

8. Last of all reduce your weight and track your BMI regularly.

Treatments by experts

You can go to physiotherapist for cure your problems. Avoid pain killers' medications.

A physio will treat you in a several way

1. Electrotherapy like long wave diathermy, interferential therapy, LASER.

2. Osteopathy and manipulation of spine to correct your faulty spine.

3. Dynamic cupping, kinesio taping, dry needling to remove hyper tender trigger points in your neck and shoulder muscles.

4. Home and office ergonomics design

5. Home self exercise protocol.

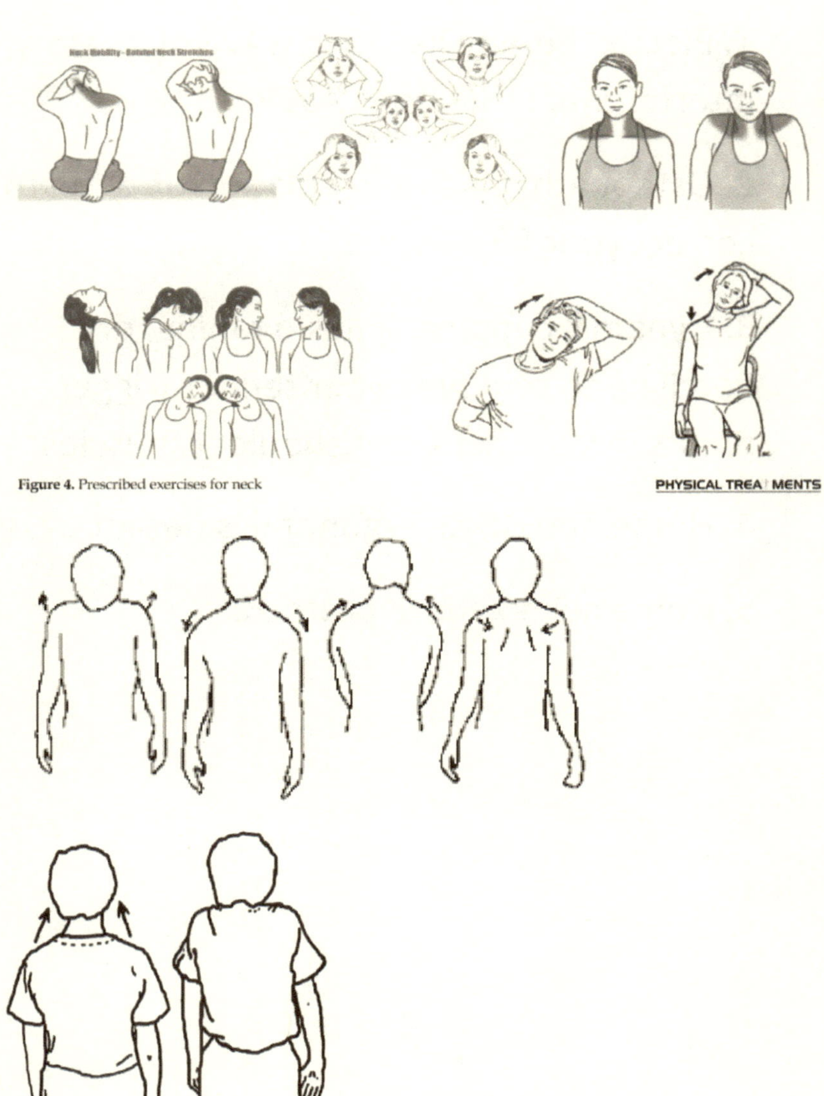

Figure 4. Prescribed exercises for neck

EXERCISES FOR TEXT NECK

www.ingramcontent.com/pod-product-compliance
Lightning Source LLC
Chambersburg PA
CBHW051133250726

48655CB00007B/3047